AGELESS
The Journal Vol 1

HH - GetFit

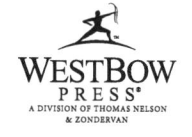

WESTBOW
PRESS®
A DIVISION OF THOMAS NELSON
& ZONDERVAN

Copyright © 2018 Heather Lynn - HHGETFIT.

All rights reserved. No part of this book may be used or reproduced by any means, graphic, electronic, or mechanical, including photocopying, recording, taping or by any information storage retrieval system without the written permission of the author except in the case of brief quotations embodied in critical articles and reviews.

Images by Blackjack Photography, HHGETFIT – Heather Lynn.

You should not undertake any diet/exercise regimen recommended in this book before consulting your personal physician. Neither the author nor the publisher shall be responsible or liable for any loss or damage allegedly arising as a consequence of your use or application of any information or suggestions contained in this book

THE HOLY BIBLE, NEW INTERNATIONAL VERSION®, NIV® Copyright © 1973, 1978, 1984, 2011 by Biblica, Inc.® Used by permission. All rights reserved worldwide.

WestBow Press books may be ordered through booksellers or by contacting:

WestBow Press
A Division of Thomas Nelson & Zondervan
1663 Liberty Drive
Bloomington, IN 47403
www.westbowpress.com
1 (866) 928-1240

Because of the dynamic nature of the Internet, any web addresses or links contained in this book may have changed since publication and may no longer be valid. The views expressed in this work are solely those of the author and do not necessarily reflect the views of the publisher, and the publisher hereby disclaims any responsibility for them.

Any people depicted in stock imagery provided by Getty Images are models, and such images are being used for illustrative purposes only. Certain stock imagery © Getty Images.

ISBN: 978-1-9736-2142-3 (sc)
ISBN: 978-1-9736-2141-6 (e)

Library of Congress Control Number: 2018902451

Print information available on the last page.

WestBow Press rev. date: 03/07/2018

Contents

Chapter 1 Me 1
Chapter 2 Let's Begin 4
Chapter 3 My Story 6
Chapter 4 Changes 10
Chapter 5 Breaking IT Down 12
Chapter 6 Moving Forward 14
Chapter 7 Change Your Mind 15
Chapter 8 Change Your Body 17
Chapter 9 Mind Body Connection 18
Chapter 10 Jumpstart Everything 21
Chapter 11 Spirit Connection 23
Chapter 12 Journaling Accountability 26
Chapter 13 Maintenance, You Time 27

I dedicate this book to my beautiful daughters Legacy and Larabea, I love you with all my heart, everything I do I do it for you.

Love, Mommy

And to my loving parents, brothers and sister thank you for always inspiring me everyday with your love and support. I love you always, Heather

1

Me

Jeremiah 29:11 For I know the plans I have for you declares the Lord plans to prosper you and not to harm you to give you a future and a hope.

I was standing in the kitchen at my house thinking how hungry I was and I begin to pace the floor thinking I will eat better today saying to myself Heather please eat better today, it was at that time I was 200 pounds.

I had just had a baby and had lost 22 pounds after the day she was born I had gained a total of 88 pounds during the pregnancy putting my weight at a whopping 222 pounds. I piled the weight on thinking I was fine that it would all vanish as soon as the baby was here. Wow was I in a dreamland the reality was before me as

I took one hard look at myself in the mirror, now don't get me wrong I was absolutely in love with my baby my little girl I lost myself in Mommy hood crying and cooing with every smile and laugh that she had made. But I took a serious look at myself and I had to be honest with Me, there were times when I was out with my family or with my friends and I was self hating myself shrinking in chairs at restaurants or in clothing shops hating myself wishing I had never gained that much weight. The reality was what it was, what have I done why did I let it go that far.

Thirteen years later I'm sitting here at my desk and I writing this book in a different city in a different home and the beautiful baby girl that I had just had is now 14 years old. I know I can't believe it time has flown! I have since had a second little baby girl she is now nine years old. I decided to sit down and pen my story and share with you my story back to health. My transformation has been radical from the inside out and has changed my life and those around me this is my story.

I grew up on the border of Mexico in Texas where the weather was warm year round the food delicious where most of my summers I would lay out by the pool and soak in the sun socializing and eating the best Mexican food you could ever eat. Delicious spices and fabulous desserts also being that it was Texas we also had delicious southern cooking, where everything is mostly fried smothered in butter and covered with flower. Delicious and beautiful desserts sweet bread, Flan Desert, fried Mexican ice cream, sopapillas soaked in honey. A dream food wise, but not health wise, being that I'm of Latino dissent, diabetes runs rampant in the Latino community as well as in my family, fatty foods laced with high salt content causing high blood pressure and high cholesterol obesity, clogged arteries and heart attacks.

2

Let's Begin

I was always a slightly chubby overweight little girl who my family regarded as shapely and big boned, during the holidays my relatives will come together we would all sit around talking and cooking and sharing about all of our fun adventures singing listening to music our talks always turn to food and how my aunt Mary was such a wonderful cook she would cook for us and make delicious meals my grandmothers would contribute and always make some amazing dishes, they would always say Heather you're just like your aunt Mary she has such a beautiful figure tiny waist big thighs full bottom. Aunt Mary was beautiful, but I didn't want much to look like aunt Mary, I very much wanted to look like my mother, thin tiny curvy ballerina dancer. My mother was so beautiful she had been a professional dancer, dancing ballet and specializing in flamenco dancing. In My eyes everything about her was perfection I idolized her. My little sister Hilary and my grandmother Beatrice favored each other in body type, thin waif look alike ballerinas, so it was hard for me at the time not being like them wanting so badly not to be curvy big boned and chunky.

3

My Story

My relationship with food as a kid was always one of love never a disoriented one, with our family we ate to be together and ate everything never counting calories or fat grams or even worrying about portion control it was always to eat what we loved, And enjoy it! It was about sharing, visiting, coming together, and loving life, loving your food, loving your environment.

It was until about the age of 12 for me we had moved from our hometown in Laredo, TX to the big city of Austin Texas where I was to go to a new private school. The move was exciting our family was thrilled new and big things were going to happen for us, my father was going to start big money deal making, it was a family adventure. I remember walking into my new private school with my school uniform fitting snug. I remember telling my mother I looked fat and felt like my skirt was tight, she assured me that I looked beautiful and sent me on my way. I walked into the new classroom feeling nervous and excited started to make new friends and adapt to my new environment. After being at school half a year I developed some good friendships and even a small crush on a boy, I remember telling one of my friends I'd liked him, one afternoon we are in the lunchroom I had overheard her telling him that I had a crush on him I remember being really embarrassed but thinking maybe he liked me, he said her? The New girl? She's fat. I was so embarrassed I ran into the bathroom. One of my friends ran after me, she said hey what's up? I said Lizzie told so and so I had a crush on him, (my crush) and he said I was fat! She said don't listen to him you're not fat. I remember looking at myself in the mirror that day as a little girl thinking yeah I am.

From that day on for the next four years I became completely aware and almost obsessed with my weight, I started turning down food when my mother cooked I also skipped meals at home parties if we went out to eat to restaurants just to lose some weight or made excuses not to eat. I remember going to summer camp and my girlfriends and I came with the camp diet we made a pact that while we were at camp we would skip breakfast we would play sports during the day we would swim all afternoon and we ate little for lunch and hardly any dinner. I can remember we were at camp for two weeks we all lost five around 10 20 pounds each when my mother picked me up from camp she gasped, she stood and looked at me and said Heather you look green are you Ok? I thought you were having fun, have you been feeling sick? I said mom I've had a blast, she says why are you looking green then? I said well we haven't really been eating that much we've been playing a lot of sports and having a lot of different activities haven't really ate much. My mom took a look at all of my friends she said all of you all look thinner, but Heather looks like she's sick Heather get in the car we're going straight to the doctor. I remember thinking I don't want to go to the doctor so I made up some excuse and we ended up going straight home.

My weight picked up and soon school started again. My girlfriends and I We talked about camp looked at all of our pictures The boys the fun the sports the swimming the tanning all the fun stuff we talked about it all including on how good we looked because we had lost so much weight and how that diet totally worked and we needed to do it again.

You know, we are so impressionable when were younger, we feel it's so important to look good that we don't take care of our health, I remember going to pool parties and my friends would say oh I've only had half an apple all day I've, only chewed gum this afternoon, I've only had a handful of this or handful of that.

And then we would all say because we've not really eaten let's order a pizza and have ice cream and will work it off tomorrow in track or in soccer or in cheerleading. We would laugh and watch movies and it was an endless cycle of binging purging starvation! All the boys were trying to grow their muscles, and taking weight gainer and all the girls were starving themselves … crazy!

All the stress that we had put on our bodies were crazy not to mention how we where messing up her menstrual cycles our hormones and by gaining and losing all the time we were slowly deteriorating ourselves. During that time my weight had plummeted I went from a healthy chunky little girl to a semi anorexic teenager all of my clothes where a 0-4 size remember my mother was small and so were my grandmothers, and my sister, so they just thought that I had baby fat and I had lost it when really I was causing harm to myself. Starvation.

The day that I was standing in the kitchen wanting to make a change after seeing my body at 200 pounds I had remembered all of these school weight memories, I had decided to make a serious change for the better but remembering binging purging starvation had led me to weight loss in the past but this could not be in my future. Healthy changes needed to happen for the better this time.

4

Changes

Dieting versus being healthy:

After I took that step forward and deciding to make that change I started reading books and looking at magazines and watching things on TV about dieting and diets, watching diet shows anything diet related, I started reading things that said eat right for your blood, what's good for you if you do this and what's good for you if you do that, I would hear people say Love your bigness love your size love yourself even though your 200 pounds and bigger. Love yourself no matter what whether you're big or small. At one point I had to stop listening and reading and watching. I felt like these were giving me mixed messages.

My baby girl was now becoming a little girl and as I was thinking as I was making all these changes to myself how is this going to affect her she was watching me, how would I explain to her with my body changing as I started to lose weight she was into princesses anything to do with Disney and she would asked me mommy do you not feel pretty do you not feel like a princess why do you want to be different I love you just away you are. I knew I needed to make healthy changes but was trying to figure out how to explain to my little girl these changes without negative connotations. I wanted her to have a healthy mindset, to grow up loving herself.

Remembering my mother, she never talked about dieting never talked about food and calories and portion control we just enjoyed our food we visit is as we ate she was and is a great cook and we enjoyed it she was naturally thin beautifully thin she never dieted she was a dancer, she would work it off in dance class. If I were to ever bring anything up like this to her she would just say there's nothing wrong with you. You're beautiful. Love yourself. You are fine. Exercise, eat, play outside, and enjoy life! There was never any talk of it. I wanted to project that to my daughter, but I also found myself at 200 pounds and needed to make some serious changes.

5

Breaking IT Down

So I broke it down I thought Ok Heather what was the size or number that you felt good in your clothes, also the weight or size that you felt the healthiest and let that connect in your mind. Then I wrote it down, and then I broke it down.

Asked myself when were you the most happy felt free ran outside played, could laugh and feel yourself, I decided to journal it, wrote it down made a mental note. Then I thought what were your favorite sports what did you enjoy doing in school what do you enjoy doing now that's good for your endurance athleticism blood pressure etc. As I thought about it I thought Ok this is not about being a size 0 this is about being healthy this is not about a number you can be a perfect size 16 like some of my friends where, and be healthy this is about health this is about healthy thinking, so I started to contemplate on what sizes had I been, when were your most healthy? What time of my life was I the most athletic eating the best, eating the right and healthy things /meals was it in high school, was it in college? I started journaling it taking a mental note reflecting and started the changes mentally.

6

Moving Forward

Moving forward mentally finding my balance. Is taking me a little while to find it completely I I've written this little book in different stages of my life journaling my thoughts in a journal along with living in different cities different homes having different jobs.

Then I was married and had my two little girls I am now a single mom, I have gone through different stages of my life and I've also been different sizes, I've been everything from a size 0 to a size 18. It's been a long difficult journey, but I've come through it Not only thinner but also stronger mentally and physically.

7

Change Your Mind

Your mind is a powerful tool you can get into mind ruts if you allow yourself to. In Texas we have a saying stinkin' thinkin' thought patterns can allow you to go into different places in your mind negativity low self-esteem depression. At the time I was going through a really hard break up I was feeling really low about myself getting into a mind rut that can flow into many areas of your life it can affect the way you look at yourself or the way you actually physically look the way you dress the way you he's at yourself, when this happens you have to take a hard look at yourself and decide to get out of that mine rut.

One of the things that have helped me is reading and quoting scriptures one of my favorites is Jeremiah 29:11 for I know the plans I have for you declares the Lord plans not to harm you but to give you a future and a hope. And I would say this to myself over and over that no matter what I was going through God did not want me to have a demise but he had planned a good future for me to rise above any negativity and weight issues I would also read positive quotes that would encourage me and give me hope on achieving my mind body goals little by little you will find yourself getting out of that rut and that way of thinking that stinkin' thinkin' and then before you know it you'll be encouraging and helping others.

As a little girl in kindergarten I was having trouble with comprehension and reading my parents had me tested and we found out I was dyslexic. Sometimes the way we are viewed by peers teachers coaches etc can be detrimental to us even early on I decided to turn those negative thoughts into positive ones it was actually pretty remarkable really, I was so young and I decided then that I did not want to be labeled like that and I wanted to change my learning and my thoughts so if I could do that with schooling I definitely could do it with these weight issues changing the way I viewed myself.

Thoughts have power change your thoughts change your life.

8

Change Your Body

Body- body mind connection:

During this time I started to reflect on my parents and their health and how my dad played football and some basketball and ran track. Very much a sports lover, I mentioned before my mother was a dancer and a cheerleader she was always very artistic by nature, these two elements have always been in my life growing up I decided to incorporate the two in my own work out routines, like my father I love track and love to run. And like my mother I love to dance and am also artistic.

9

Mind Body Connection

Working out:

In the beginning at 200 pounds I started walking slowly around my neighborhood I would walk my block briskly, I would get my heart rate up, If I felt it was a little high I would back down and would slow down I would do this for about a month. As soon as I feel my energy lifting, and I could do a little more, for another month I would do a walk jog, as soon as I feel that working, energy rising, I would add or intern make that a jog, I would do that for a month, and then I would turn my jogging into a full-blown run. I lost about 15 to 20 pounds this way along with changing my diet started to eat cleaner cut out fast food, sodas, and ate very little sweets. No cookies, white bread, cakes etc.

I did this for a while until the wait wasn't coming off. I decided to join a gym looked around started googling, and through one of my friends heard about a private gym that her friends had. I had saved up some money and decided to put down $2000 hired two trainers and joined their Boot Camp, and weightlifting classes, I did this for about six months day in day out, it took about eight months for me to see a difference, a lot of blood sweat and tears, I was one of the biggest ones there starting at 195 pounds. It was a great work out pushing through obstacles, I lost the bulk of my weight with this type of work out I did a lot of lunges, squats, running lines, kettle bell swing's, timed runs, push-ups, crunches, all at high intensity one hour sessions at 5 AM and at 6 PM I did this for a period of eight months and lost 50 pounds doing it this way. I logged on my IG page and my Twitter Account for all to see I was so proud I was gradually losing.

I also decided to incorporate Zumba, being that my mother was a dancer and danced throughout all of her pregnancies and most of my life we always had music and dance in our home and I myself took dance classes, I needed this in my life and Zumba was a great way to do that for me, find movement with sweating and a workout routine. I loved it so much I got certified as a Zumba instructor. I continue to this day to love Zumba!

Also I added Yoga, Hot yoga, was a great way of working out I found it to warm up my muscles and lengthened my limbs and stretched me out after mornings at Boot Camp, and weightlifting, yoga was a great way to sooth my muscles at the end of the day not to mention to help me sweat and clear out the toxins from my body.

10

Jumpstart Everything

Last but not least – weightlifting:

I completely love weightlifting it has helped sculpt my muscles and tone up the loose skin from losing weight, When I was 200 pounds I remember looking at magazines that had bodybuilders on the cover with beautiful physiques and I remember thinking I would love to be like that I would love to be a bodybuilder, and thought one day I will! I have come this far I had already lost 65 pounds and was gaining great momentum from all these different workout routines. Friends Family and people started stopping me on the street asking me what I was doing, my friends said Heather you've lost so much weight you look so good and happy what are you doing? Or I would have strangers say you're so smiley and your skin glows what's your secret. And I would tell them about different workout routines I was doing to shed the weight, but in all actuality it wasn't just the weight I was shedding, I was shedding years of stuff, bad patterns not only in eating, but my thinking, also going through a really hard break up with my marriage, could've sent me in a deep depression but thinking positive, feeling positive, quoting scriptures and getting in tune with my spirit. Has literally changed my life for the better and I continue to grow and evolve into who God wants me to be. Mostly doing my workouts indoor outdoor with my walk runs small jogs full-blown runs my cardio is very important I always try to find time to squeeze it in, I eventually bought a treadmill so I could do my cardio in doors as well at the gym I would also use the elliptical or the stair climber as workouts those are really beneficial as well but I still prefer to go outside overall and walk it out, work it out, I feel it so important to wake up our brains and feel the sunshine and to get that vitamin D that we need. I have two brothers who have companies that deal with the outdoors and their motto is "enjoy this creation that we live on and go outside"! Use it to clear your thoughts and to refresh your mind it helps you jumpstart and start over.

11

Spirit Connection

Mind body spirit connection:

Bringing it all to a close, looking back at my childhood and all the love, food, family, love of the outdoors. Remembering my childhood and how fun it was, my father who is such a brilliant Man, who taught me so much on how to think and be careful what I say. Those are powerful tools he would say. His father was a pastor and a missionary to Mexico they taught him the fundamental principles about speech and how to help others and to be positive and to love others

Unconditionally and to give by giving you receive. He also suffered from dyslexia like me and made himself from nothing to something working as a car salesman, cleaning trains, to becoming an adventure capitalist, buying and selling real estate, property oil and hotels traveling the world. He has taught me so much, everything from how to stand how to talk to others, even fashion, he has such a great sense of fashion. Beautiful clothes, He and my Mother loved Beautiful vacations loved Hawaii traveled to Paris to visit and to shop in private jets living in beautiful homes and driving beautiful cars. But most importantly loving people and treating everyone equally. After traveling to beautiful destinations we could go eat with the taco vendor in a hole in the wall place and laugh and visit for hours where my parents taught us never to judge people places or things, mindset is everything, work ethic is important no matter what your background or circumstances are. My dad would say, if you take this with you you can live anywhere in the world positivity loving others, being kind, That is everything! My family instilled this in me at a Young age as well as my siblings I intern instill this in my own children.

When you incorporate all of that with positive thinking and successful workouts it's easy to incorporate the next step, "Your Spirit"

For me that starts with a God factor, growing up my relationship with God was and is everything and has been everything he's my anchor my foundation with him I am everything without him I am nothing.

I attended Raima Bible College and it's really strong on the spoken word so I try to speak the word of God over my life so it goes into my spirit and it creates a strong root of faith love and hope. I feel without these fruits of the spirit we crumble, everybody needs hope to continue towards tomorrow, we need love to thrive, and we need faith to grow and reach towards our next levels.

I challenge you to change your mindset to cleanse your heart and cleanse your mind of any negative thoughts of unworthiness or in adequacy's thanking God for your day rather than filling your day with useless busy stuff or complaining or any negativity or bad language.

I guarantee you once you start this it becomes so contagious to yourself and to others that your environment will be filled with joy and happiness and change.

12

Journaling Accountability

Overall maintenance:

I recommend for overall maintenance that you check yourself, that you journal, meditate take time out for you, whether you are a male or a female, take time out and spend time doing things you love, whether that's hanging out with friends, going to the mall, going out to eat, going to the movies, for me it's getting a manicure and a pedicure or massage and just chilling out or maybe even going shopping, but it keeps you in check with yourself in caring for yourself don't ever lose yourself. It's so easy in this day and age with media, things that are going on in the world, that we forget us, we always put our families first, or churches, work, friends, businesses, let's not forget ourselves. We only have one life Lets live it to the fullest!

13

Maintenance, You Time

Finding your outlet:

For me that was music, music has always been my life my first love, as a professional singer singing on TBN and doing cover work for Sony Latin in Miami and Zuma records, Music was always an outlet to feel free to find a place I could go to and enjoy my passion. Find your passion find your outlet. For me it's also health and fitness.

Find your health find your passion Finding an outlet will be an added bonus for you it will give you even more reason to thrive and have hope towards those greater goals.

Diet & Recipes

Clean eating:

Diet is so very important I would say that it's probably 90% of your weight loss and health healing. There's a saying, "Abs are made in the kitchen." So true! With all of my workouts and everything I've done it's a combination of everything together that creates balance and makes everything flow smoothly. This is what I did:

I ate every 2 to 3 hours 5 to 6 meals a day. It's helped me speed up my metabolism. At first it feels like you're gaining weight, it did for me anyway. I put on a little bit of weight as I started my weight loss journey. Along with workouts, I seemed to bulk up at first but as I kept on with it eventually my body balanced out and started losing weight.

The diet plan that I have here to lose weight is a meat eaters diet; I am now incorporating other options of protein then animal protein into my diet. I am now adding more plant/vegetarian-based options similar to the ones below. There are so many options out there, in organic vegetables, beans, lentils, etc. that can offer you lots of protein and taste much the same as animal protein. The options below I have tried myself and they are delicious.

Keep in mind: if you have peanut allergies instead of one spoonful of peanut butter with your organic apple or in your protein shakes/smoothies substitute organic cashew butter or sunflower seed butter. These are delicious substitutes!

Eat and enjoy!

Breakfast:

Three egg whites
1-cup spinach
1-teaspoon chopped onion to taste
Cracked pepper
Himalayan Pink salt
One English muffin (toasted)

Two hours later Midmorning snack:

Protein shake - strawberry or birthday cake flavor (My Favorites!)
Make sure it's low in carbs, low in sugar, and high in protein. Pick a brand of your choice.
Three hours later – Lunch:
6-Ounces organic grilled chicken breast

Mixed organic green salad
Half cup of baby organic tomatoes
Organic shredded carrots (half cup)
Organic spray olive oil (spray lightly over tossed salad)
2-teaspoons of organic balsamic vinegar.

Three hours later – Snack:

One organic apple
1-tablespoon of organic peanut butter

Two hours later – Dinner:

6-ounce organic salmon, chicken or steak (grilled or baked)
1-cup organic brown rice
Organic Spinach green leafy side salad
1/2 cup dried organic cranberries
Organic olive oil spray (spray all over salad)
2-tablespoons of organic balsamic vinegar.

For vegetarians:

In place of 6-ounce Salmon, Steak, Chicken you can do:
6-ounce Organic Veggie burger patties
6-ounce Organic Veggie chicken patties,
6 ounce Organic Veggie fajita chicken
6-ounce Tofu burgers.
6-ounce organic black bean burgers
You can find these at many health food grocery stores.

Two hours later – Snack (Something low in carbs):

Like half a cup of almonds
1-teaspoon peanut butter

Drinks:

Organic Green tea
Organic Black tea (Brewed – drink cold or hot)
Water (Lots and lots of water)
You can't drink enough water. It flushes out the toxins and it is good for your skin.
I drink water all day throughout the day!

To jumpstart your system and your body, make sure to find a good overall body cleanse you can get these at any health grocery store's. It'll help jumpstart your system and your diet. Once you do this I say then get into your workout regimen, then start your Organic eating and diet. This should help your overall well-being and also you will be on your way to losing weight and regaining your health back.

Also make sure you take a good multivitamin This way you won't feel depleted of anything once you start your workouts, if you have any questions I recommend you ask your doctor before starting any diet or consuming any type of vitamins.

You will be well on your way to losing weight.

Recipes - my favorite fast easy recipes-

Recipe 1

Organic shredded carrot salad:
One package shredded organic carrots
Organic olive oil spray- I spray it until the shredded carrots are nice and coated organic balsamic vinegar likely drizzled, Himalayan pink salt, cracked fresh black pepper, to taste, half cup organic dried cranberries, 1 cup shredded parmesan cheese or one cup crumbled blue cheese. Ready to eat.

Recipe 2

Avocado salad:
4 or 5 large organic avocados scooped and pitted
Avocados Chopped and mashed.
One large organic lime cut and squeeze into the avocado mixture.
1-cup chopped organic cilantro
1-cup chopped organic tomato
Half cup chopped organic red onion
Pink Himalayan salt for taste.
Cracked fresh black pepper for taste.
Eat as a snack or as a side with any meal.

Recipe 3

Organic gluten free protein pancakes:

You can buy organic gluten-free pancake mix at any healthy grocery store in your area.

Create the pancake mixture like it reads on the box, and then add one scoop of your favorite protein powder put one scoop in the mixture and you will have delicious organic gluten-free protein pancakes. Make and ready to serve.

Topping- flavored yogurt. Then add fresh organic strawberries raspberries or

blueberries.

Or you can add 100% organic maple syrup,

Or half cup melted butter mixed with warmed honey drizzle on top. You can also add organic crumbled walnuts on top sprinkle with cinnamon and one dollop of Low-fat organic Cool Whip on top.

Recipe 3

Baked sweet potato:
(Great as a side dish or as a snack)
Two large organic sweet potatoes
Purple or orange (the organic purple ones are much sweeter then the orange ones)
Bake in the oven at 375 until tender,
1-teaspoon of organic butter
One teaspoon of organic brown sugar
Sprinkle organic powdered cinnamon to taste
Cracked Himalayan pink salt to taste
1/2 cup organic gluten-free marshmallows to taste
Once all melted and baked it's ready to eat.

Recipe 4

Mango and Pineapple:
Peeled and sliced three mangoes
Cut a half of a pineapple make into wedges.
Arranged nicely on the plate, sprinkle organic chili lime seasoning salt on top.
Delicious little snack that is sweet and spicy.

Closing prayer:

I want to give you the opportunity for you to accept Jesus Christ as your personal savior he's the one that makes all my blessings flow he is the one who is cured me of all my diseases by knowledge and wisdom giving me understanding on everything. Pray this with me: you can say this out loud or you can whisper it to yourself or in your heart.

Jesus, I thank you and I give you all the glory and all the honor for my life I thank you that you have introduced me to this book I receive all the knowledge and all the understanding that was shared I take it with me on my daily journey and I give you the glory and the honor for my life I ask for you to come into my heart and to change me and to make me a new vessel and to give me peace and to give me faith and grace and hope to handle my life and all that comes with it and the journey you have for me in Jesus name I pray amen.

Thank you for reading my book and giving me the opportunity to share my story with you and my journey

I hope it is blessed you I hope your journey will be as transforming as mine has been I hope it touched your heart …

Thank you,

Heather

Gallery Section

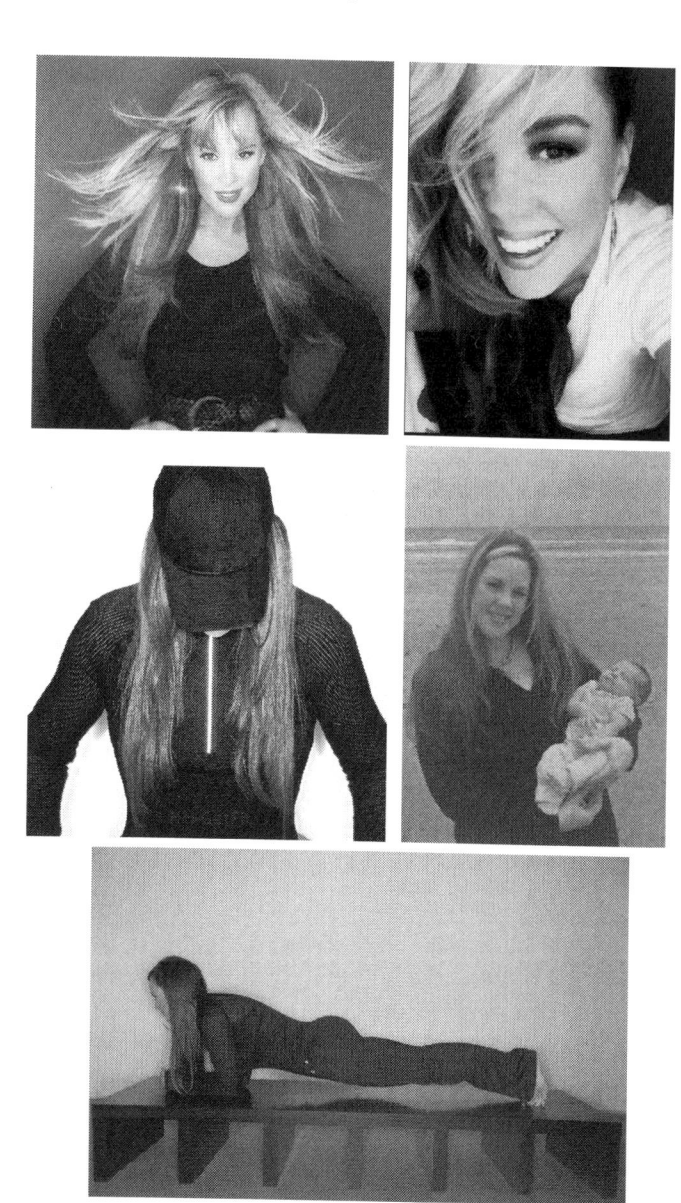

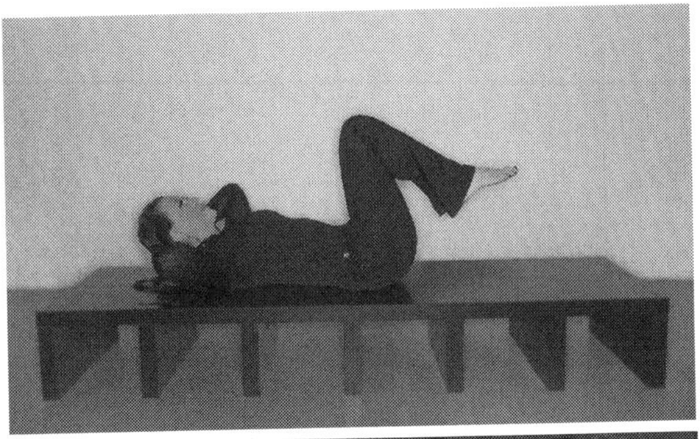

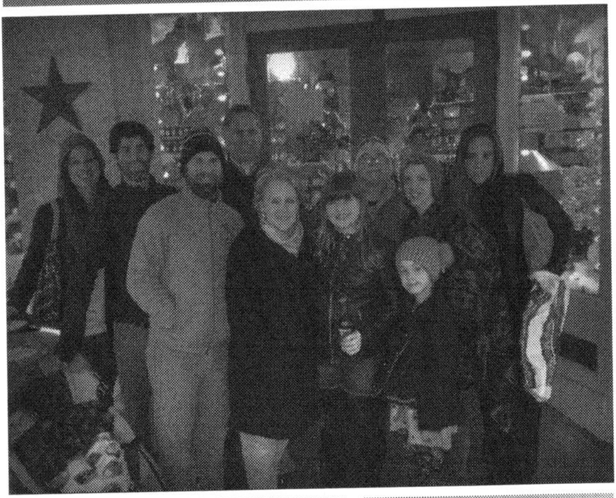

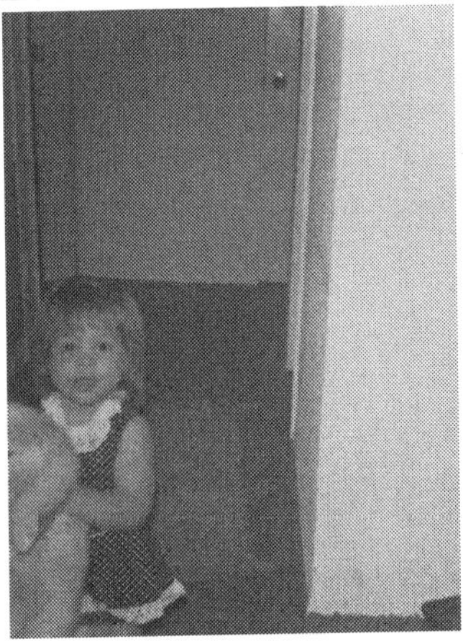

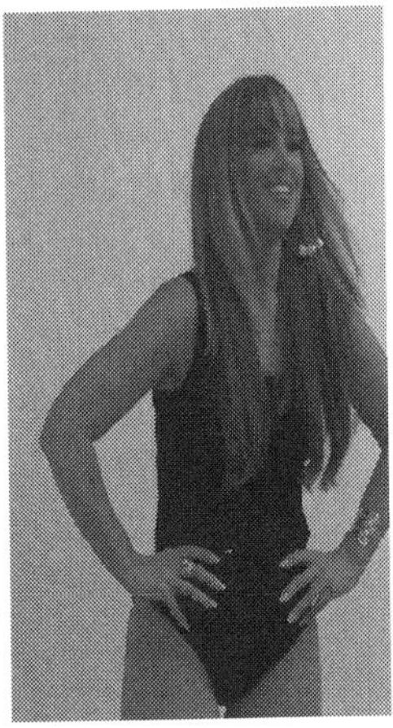

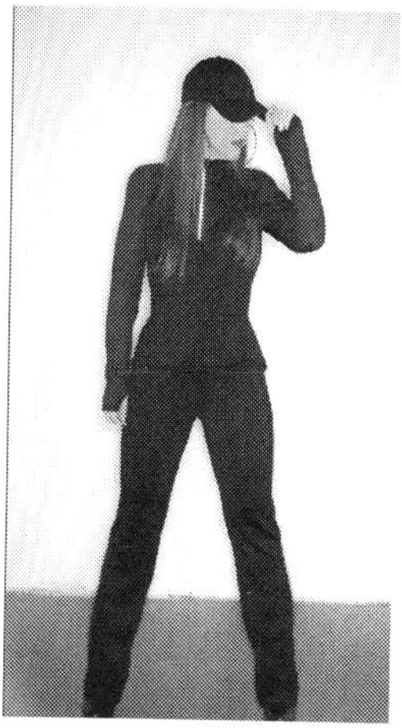

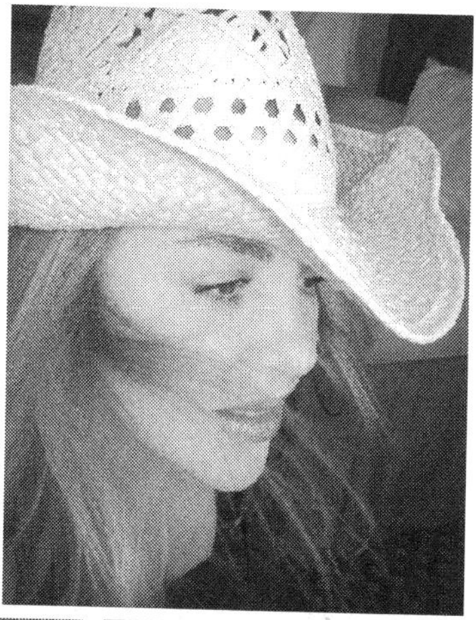

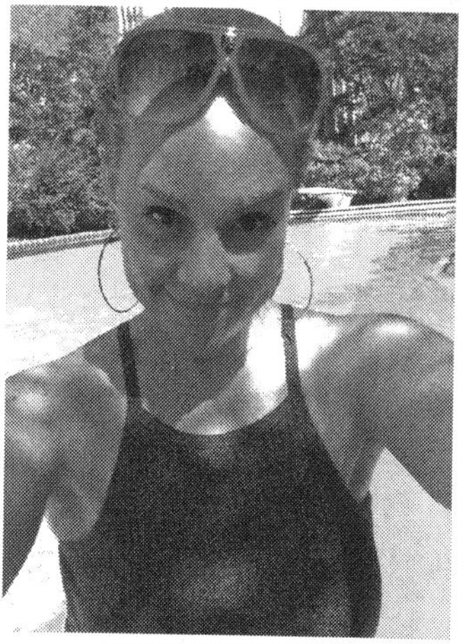

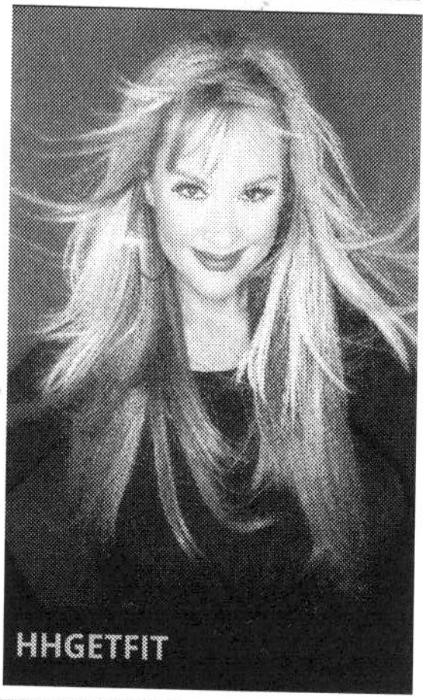
HHGETFIT

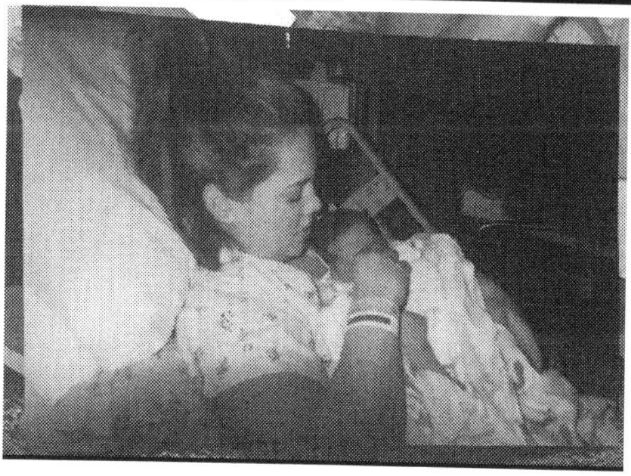

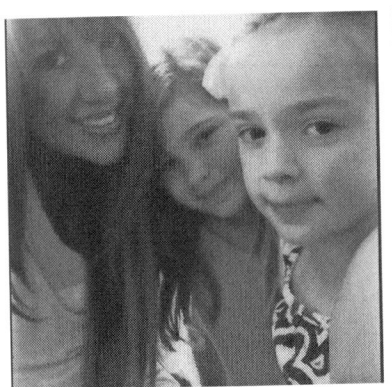

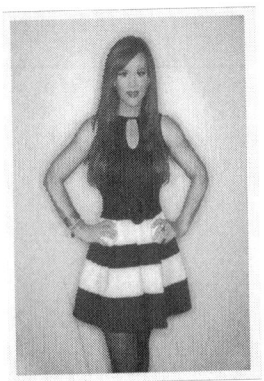

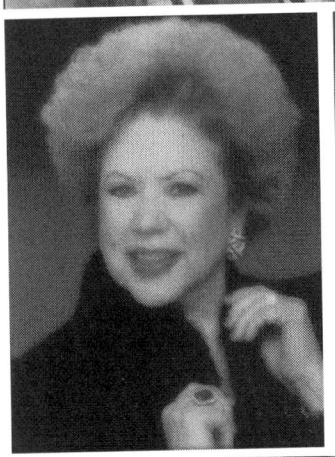

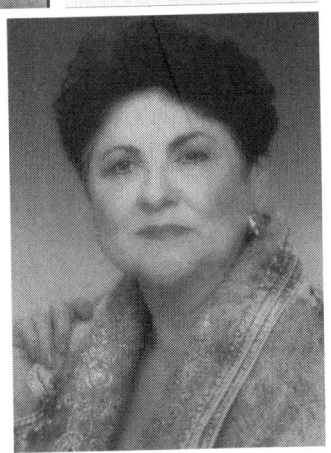

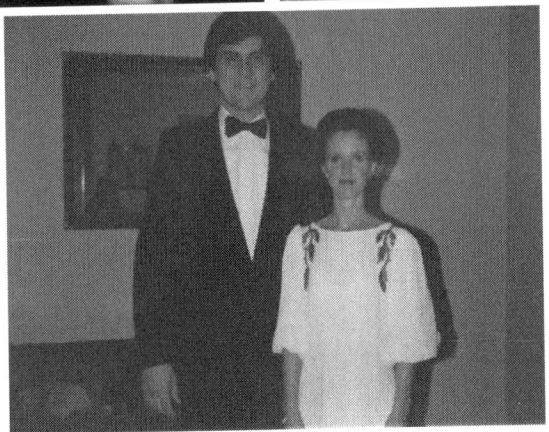

Made in the USA
Lexington, KY
04 May 2018